ASHLE

GET $HIT DONE

IT'S TIME TO GET OFF THE COUCH...

Copyright © 2016 by Ashley Mathieu
All Rights Reserved.

Images © BigStock, Ashley Matiheu

ISBN 978-1-5301-9088-1

CONTENTS

INTRODUCTION 5

Chapter 1: Ask yourself WHY 9
Chapter 2: Taking out the trash 19
Chapter 3: Get active & Create the schedule 25
Chapter 4: The Help 34
Chapter 5: Fueling your body for success 43
Chapter 6: Supplements – Do you need them? . 56
Chapter 7: Stretch yourself 62
Chapter 8: Avoid the Media & Hype 67
Chapter 9: I'll shut up now 72

Acknowledgements 75
Ashley's Picks 79

INTRODUCTION

I want to thank you and give you a *high five* for reaching out and buying my book. This book contains no bull shit strategies on how to get healthy, be stronger physically and mentally, build confidence, be happy and understand how to live a balanced lifestyle for YOURSELF. I put this book together by gathering my own personal experiences with career, health, fitness and years of coaching clients to a healthier lifestyle. Hearing clients struggle, complain and nag about not being able to lose weight, handling personal issues and other lifestyle stresses, I decided to reach out to the rest of the world with this book. I was someone who grew up with struggles as a kid at home, in school, with myself, in the hospital dealing with health issues for many years, emotional and physical abuse, along with a lack of desire to step foot in the workplace. The one main thing that helped me through it all was keeping active. Having an outlet to release any stress, anxiety or frustration. Being able to have a focus on soccer, hockey, kickboxing, Muay Thai and lifting weights helped me escape what was going on around me. I can't thank my coaches enough for that. No matter the mood I was in or what I was going through, they were always there to push me and lend an ear. My parents who probably wanted to slap me around sometimes and gave me tough love. Can't say I was a saint of a child!

I ended up leaving my career in the Government in 2010. I wanted to be happy, live life and help others do the same. I let everything build up over a few years. I finally had the courage to say enough was enough. Fall of 2010 I said the famous two words, "I Quit" via email in the passenger seat of my buddies car, tethering the internet from his phone to my laptop. I can tell you the largest font for hotmail was 30. That's as large as I could go when I wrote, "I QUIT" in my email. From that, I continued on my 2 week road trip to the east coast. Scariest but best decision I ever made. I didn't tell my parents or friends for at least a week. I knew they would think I was crazy, stupid or just straight up out of my mind for quitting a job with benefits, pension and something that was considered safe. At the end of the day, I didn't give two shits. Life was far more important to me than steady pay. I wanted to live life happy and get back to being myself. I no longer wanted to be miserable and potentially never appreciate my pension. With my luck I'd be in my grave before I got it! Sounds kind of morbid, but it's the truth. Life is short. You never know when your expiry date will kick in.

I understand how important it is to tell the negatives in life to take a hike, live every day like it's your last, go after what makes you happy and not let shit get in the way of your success and health. I've been that person who dove head first into food as an emotional support, gained weight and didn't care. Who lived every day in the gym to avoid everything else. Who stayed under a rock to avoid society, to be alone. Who at some point didn't give a shit what happened around me or to me. I've been there, done that. Never again. Now I want to help others get out of the ruts, out from under their rocks, out of their heads and into life by keeping the pedal to the floor. Again, life is too short. Why wait until it's too late? Why wait until the doctor gives you bad news? Why wait until you are cripple and in pain? Why wait until your rope has run out? Why wait until you hit rock bottom?

WHY. ARE. YOU. WAITING.

Society is far too confused about what is considered healthy, how to be healthy and how to live your life. My life lessons and tips are straight forward. I hope to give you a realistic approach in dealing with fitness, nutrition and lifestyle. No more lies. No more sugar coating. No more negative self talk. No more thinking you can't do something. No more living a life where you feel there is no escape. Just straight forward talk, zero bull shit and helpful information to get you to YOUR goals! All the information in this book is exactly what I did to get where I am.

I will make a couple things clear... If you decide after you read this book to make a change, be prepared that it may not be easy for you and it may take a lot more time than you want. It took my 5 years to get to where I am today. A zero bull shit, goal driven and confident entrepreneur. One who gets up every day wanting to make people laugh, educate and push people to rise above the bull shit that surrounds them. BOOM! *Enter knuckles here*

Thanks again. I hope you enjoy the next few hours of your life reading my randomness. And... Be warned. I do drop some 'shit' bombs in here. If you bought this book, you clearly don't get offended easily. If you were given this book, well... I warned you.

Ashley Mathieu

CHAPTER 1:
ASK YOURSELF **WHY**

First and for most, you need to understand **WHY** you are doing something. If you start a project, no matter the subject, you need to understand **WHY** you are doing it. When I wanted to quit my career, I wrote down exactly **WHY** I wanted to leave. This helped me understand that it was more than disliking a certain someone in the office. It really pointed out more and opened the doors to further conversation with myself as to **WHY**. I wrote down on a piece of paper, "If I died tomorrow, would I be happy? Would I have regrets?" The answer to that question was, no I wouldn't be happy and yes I would have regrets. I asked myself...Why? I wouldn't be happy because I was angry at where my career had gone. I wasn't doing what truly made me happy. The negative environment changed who I was. I was no longer the happy, fun, outgoing person my friends knew me to be. I was negative and defensive. I was constantly looking over my shoulder and wondering when the next random act of shit was going to happen. My personal life took a hit because I wasn't happy with myself, which bled into my relationships. Who wants a partner who constantly bitches about work? One of my regrets was letting the workplace situations eat away at me, get the better of me and change who I was as a person. I don't regret having the career or going through what I went through in my early 20's. I met some really good people and some I am still in contact with until this day. If it wasn't for the situations I faced, people I met, I wouldn't be where I am today and I sure as hell wouldn't be as strong mentally or emotionally. It was at the age of 27 where I realized I was no longer going to be scared or treated a certain way.

UNDERSTANDING YOUR WHY IS NOT ONLY POWERFUL, BUT IMPORTANT.

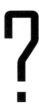

GET SHIT DONE

Let's grab a pen. Get out a book or a piece of paper. I want you to write your name on the paper. Congratulations, you can spell your name. If you haven't written your name, shame on you. Second, let's write the date down. OK, now you have a piece of paper with your name and date written down... We are off to a great start! (Can you tell I'm a sarcastic ass yet?) I want you to write down your name and date so that in a few months, you can go back and read everything. YOU decided on this date that YOU were going to address issues and make changes. Hold yourself accountable.

I want you to write down **WHY** you bought this book. If there is more than one reason, write them down. After you are done that, I want you to write down **WHY** you gave those reasons for purchasing this book. Let me say it again, the power of the word **WHY** is powerful. You can find out so many things just by using that one word. Start by using it on yourself and don't be afraid of your own thoughts or answers that may pop up. That's the whole point of this exercise. If you don't understand **WHY** you are doing something, then **WHY** are you doing it?! I know it can be scary to take skeletons out of the closet, but if we don't deal with them now, they will eventually come to bite you in the ass later on.

Write this stuff down before moving forward. Please and thank you.

Moving on... Now I am going to ask you **WHAT** your goals are. Let's make one thing clear, your goals need to be REALISTIC! Creating unrealistic goals will set you up for disaster. When creating your goals, I want you to think of important things in your life you want to accomplish. If I tell you to create goals in a year from now, you will most likely fluff it off and not do it. I am not saying that to be a jerk, I'm saying this because I see it daily. People come up with health and fitness goals in a year, then that year comes... Oh look... You gave up because you lacked accountability and stopped giving a shit. Start small with one goal at a time. Don't get me wrong, you can have an outlook of what you want in the future... But in order to get there, it's the initial goals that set up the foundation.

I knew my goal was to be an entrepreneur, but needed to learn. I was heading into a new industry full time. I left my condo downtown Ottawa for the basement of my parents' house. Emotional eating made awesome by mom's cooking! My goal was to get hired by a big box club and get out of the basement in a year. I gave myself a timeline.

I knew I needed to learn different training styles, how the business worked and how things were run. I shadowed other trainers, took classes that I wouldn't usually take and made it a point to talk to everyone. I wanted to break things down to better understand not only the industry but also what clients want. Once I accomplished that, the next goal was to set up my own shop. I did just that 8 months later, setting up shop in a private training studio in south Ottawa where I was now a full time entrepreneur, focused on my own brand (www.ashleymathieu.com). I was happy, excited, broke, motivated and finally turning back into my old self. I was eating better, exercising almost every day, my attitude was MUCH more positive, got my competitive edge back and had tunnel vision on being the best person I could be. I was working alongside other independent trainers who all had their own style. We all helped one another out. We supported one another. I learned what it was like to be on my own as an entrepreneur. Paying rent, marketing, how to handle feedback, what it was like when business was slow, how to get creative and see the positive in every negative situation. Business went well and I was in my own place exactly one year after moving back home.

    A year after being in the studio, I looked long term. What did I want to do? I love training, love helping people, love educating... Why not own a gym?! A few years back I was lucky to have a franchise owner of Snap Fitness help sponsor me when I was competing in kick boxing. I thought of Allister right away and remember what he told me. Also another person who quit a career for health. (Thanks Allister)

So, off I went to research more about franchises. During this time the universe decided to send a man into my life. This guy's name is Mike. We actually met because I made a bunch of complaints about the new property I was in. Ha! After we both discovered our love for Ferrari, that was it. We had a professional relationship and built a close friendship. In 2013, I signed on the dotted line with Anytime Fitness with my friend and business partner. Boom.

AND BACK TO THE CHAPTER...

I am constantly looking for new goals in the gym. That's what keeps me going. For weight lifting, I look at a weight I have never lifted before and tell myself I am going to lift it in a certain time frame. I know how I am going to program my training in order to lift it. Example, I was staring at the 60lbs dumbbells sitting on the rack. I had never attempted a flat bench dumbbell press with 60lbs in each hand before. **WHY** would I want to lift them?

GET $HIT DONE

Because I never have. That's **WHY**! I looked over at DJ (one of the best trainers a club can have) and said, "I'm going to make those dumbbells my bitch at least once". The next week I tried. Nope, no dice. Not a chance. I even filmed it and posted it on social media. I showed the world I 'failed'. Gave me more drive to lift them the next week. The next week rolls around, called DJ over to spot me and get Vishaal (pretty cool member at the club) to film it. Sure as hell do I not press them! I was so pumped I went for a second rep which went up half way and that's about it! The feeling of pressing those 60lbs dumbbells for the first time, even for one rep, was awesome! I had never done it before. Set goals and SMASH them! If it doesn't work out the first time, try again! The only failure is you NOT trying.

UNDERSTANDING YOUR WHY ACCOMPANIED WITH GOALS IS A PRETTY POWERFUL THING.

Some examples of simple goal setting:

- *Short:* Set up a short term goal within 6 weeks. It can be a weight loss goal of going down a notch on your belt, cardio goal of being able to run a couple more minutes without stopping or cutting down on a bad habit. Example of that could be trying to quit smoking, going from 1 pack a day to half a pack in 6 weeks. Perhaps it's just to make yourself active 2 times a week. Update your resume? Apply to different positions? Create a business plan?

- *Medium:* Next we want to think about a goal you can tackle in 6 months. Maybe get into those old jeans, lose 20lbs or be able to run 5km (or Miles if you're American!). Hey, maybe it's simply STAYING the same weight that you are at and avoiding the fluctuation.

- *Long Term:* Last is the big 1 year goal. This is a big one because when you smash this, it feels like a massive accomplishment! If you're in this for a weight loss journey, make sure you have a target goal for overall weight loss. If it's lifestyle change, try for 1 year being active for a minimum of 3 times a week. It can be as awesome as in 1 year you want to have gone from the couch, to living life to its fullest by having a balanced diet, regular exercise regime, creating positivity and being strong! Maybe it's to get a new job. New career. GET IT!

GET SHIT DONE

I want you to imagine yourself completing these goals. How do you feel? Why do you feel this way? Try and put yourself in the time frame where you are accomplishing all the goals you just listed. If you don't feel all kinds of awesome, GET SOME NEW GOALS! You should be ****ing jazzed right up! GET EXCITED! BE EXCITED! You should be yelling WOO and scaring the shit out of someone right now!

All of these are just ideas from me to you. Make realistic goals. This book is to help YOU get where you want to be physically and mentally. Don't do what others THINK you should do. This is your life. It's your body. Your mentality. I am here to get YOU up and kicking ass for YOURSELF! Understood? Yes? Cool... Moving on.

"WHEN YOUR INNER STRENGTH BECOMES SUPERIOR, YOUR EVERYDAY BECOMES EASIER..."

– ASHLEY MATHIEU

CHAPTER 2:
TAKING OUT THE TRASH

In this chapter I am going to get you to take out the trash! What do I mean? In the previous chapter we came up with goals. However, sometimes when we have an objective, things like to get in the way. Some classic obstacles that my clients have had to overcome are:

- Family not approving of the lifestyle change. They think it's a phase, not realistic or dumb.
- Spouse not supporting your goals.
- Friends being negative or sabotaging your nutrition changes.
- Little support in the work environment.
- Getting caught up in the media with new 'miracle' weight loss pill, diet or workout.

- Negative self talk.
- Comparing yourself to others.
- Negative personal life (relationships).

TIP 1: Here's the thing. If you have someone around you who does not support you going after a healthy and stress free lifestyle for yourself, it's probably better you don't have them around. Think about it, if your friends, family and spouse care about you and love you, they will stick by whatever decision you make. No matter if they like it or not. If they are negative towards your decision to change for the better, they may need to be educated on **WHY** you chose to change as they simply might not understand. If they don't care to understand, then it may be time to leave them at the curb or simply ignore them. Sometimes you just have to do you! Stop messing around with your physical and mental health. Remember, this is for YOU! Putting up with other people's trash isn't your responsibility. Straight up. (Yeah, I went gangster there...) Why waste your energy on dealing with someone else's BS when you could be taking that energy and utilizing it on yourself? Side note. Not all criticism should be taken as negative. They could be trying to give you a different view after you ranted;)

GET $HIT DONE

TIP 2: Surround yourself with people who support you. The more support you have around you, the better frame of mind you will be in. This is very important for those of you who have become negative about yourself. Having positivity around you will only help your positive outlook. If you need to speak with a therapist or some sort of third party, then do it! There is no shame in that. There could be a lot of things going on that you don't recognize and need a third party to point out. Our minds are our own worst enemies. We spend a lot of time thinking instead of doing. Start paying attention to how much you live in your own head, the constant self talk, comparing, putting yourself down etc... Bet you it's far more common than you think. Next time you catch yourself saying you CAN'T do something, picture me standing in front of you with arms crossed saying, "Get Shit Done".

TIP 3: During your journey, you will hit walls. It's your positive and driven mindset that will get you through it. Do NOT compare your progress or goals to others. Your body is not the same as the person next to you. You have created a goal for yourself that may be similar to someone else, however the path to get there might be very different. DO NOT get caught up on what you see on the television or what you read in a magazine. Supplement companies make up a multimillion dollar industry. They have fancy labels and fun wording to get your attention. Cutting corners by taking pills and powders can lead to more health issues than you think, even more so when you take something your body doesn't agree with. So before you start loading yourself up with foreign shit, understand YOUR body first! You can't reformat your body like a computer. You can't walk into a store and exchange yourself. Learn how your body functions like how you take the time to read instructions before you build that IKEA cabinet!

TIP 4: Get rid of the negativity around you. Make sure your outlook on what you want is pure. Have all your ducks in a row in terms of the life situations you can change or adjust. Put up positive affirmations on your desktop background, replace the background on your phone, swap out 'nothing' pictures on your wall with positive quotes and try to see a positive in a negative situation. If you can't see a positive in the negative situation, then tell it to take a hike! I have what I call the 'f**k it' switch. If something is sucking my energy and it's not worth it, I say, "f**k it'! Move on! What is the point of wasting your energy on useless shit? NONE! If it doesn't directly affect you, leave it. Suck up your ego, walk away, learn to laugh and dance like you're Ellen. That's at least how I dance...

GET SHIT DONE

So to rehash what I spoke about earlier in the chapter, there is nothing wrong with acknowledging you might need professional help for whatever situation is causing you a mental shit storm. Sometimes you can't do everything by yourself. It's OK to ask for help! I'll tell you from a personal stand point when I decided to change my direction, I realized I was headed down a path of self destruction working in an environment that was highly toxic. I couldn't speak with many people at work because I was worried it would lead to a mud slide of shit. I escaped to my family members where I felt safe and not judged. Eventually I went to see a third party to get some insight from someone who didn't know me. I found this a big help. They weren't biased. They gave me different views, listened, answered questions and took massive weight off my shoulders. I was able to see a different side to things I couldn't before because I was blinded by a constant negative mind frame. All this helped me map my plan of action (kind of) and then at 2am on that Thursday morning, I quit my job and started my new journey in 2012 where I took my talent and passion for health and fitness to a whole other level! I quit a 'safe' job in the Government to be a full time entrepreneur. Scary as shit, but well worth it! Side note, it is still scary as shit!

"WITH THE NEW DAY COMES
NEW STRENGTHS AND NEW THOUGHTS"

− ELEANOR ROOSEVELT

CHAPTER 3:
GET ACTIVE & CREATE THE SCHEDULE

You can always say, "I'm going to start this week" and then when the week is done you realized you did absolutely nothing! This is where the schedule comes in handy. It's finding those time gaps you never realized you had. The number one complaint I hear from people is, "I don't have time". That's a load of crap! Let's be real. If you can't find the time, look for it. Simple. Enough with the excuses. As we covered in the last chapter, ask for help if you need it.

If you are starting to get off the couch, let's start with 2-3 days where we get you moving. I want you to start by writing down the times you work on a calendar. Try and use a calendar that's easy to read. If you live off the calendar on your phone, use your phone. If you need something bigger, head to a store and get one of those massive desk top calendars. Put that sucker to use. Maybe you love cats and want to use a cat calendar. Whatever. Put it up in a place where you see it daily, like the fridge or maybe a cork board in the kitchen.

- Write down the days you work
- Write down any family activities you have to tackle
- Write down any plans already made

I want you to see the gaps. If you are the type of person to get up early, set the morning aside for yourself. Maybe you like your sleep and prefer an afternoon or evening workout. Whatever, just pick a time that works best for YOU.

Again, do NOT do what someone else tells you to do. I personally hate working out early in the morning. I am a straight up useless tit. Never liked it. Actually, scratch that. I liked it, "this one time" when I had gone through a break up and enjoyed getting up early to walk along the water. That was my serenity. But since I got over that, I haven't liked mornings! Fast forward… I have terrible workouts in the morning because I would much rather sleep. I make the time in the early afternoons or evenings because that's what works for me. Not only is that usually the time of day where I have the most energy but it's also the less hectic time of day for me.

GET $HIT DONE

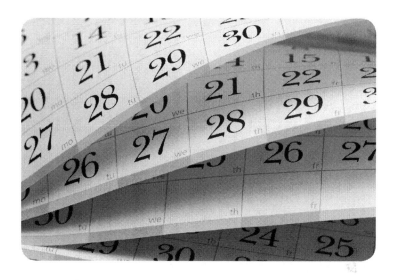

- **BRIGHT EYED AND BUSHY TAILED:** You are the best people to deal with! I swear! You guys are up super early before the world rotates! This makes getting shit done pretty easy. You're already up sitting on the couch watching the news or reading the paper. Mine as well use that time to get your workout in! Can be as simple as heading out for a 30 minute walk with the dog, easy exercises from home or if you have the time, drive to the gym near your house for a workout... Like perhaps Anytime Fitness (shameless plug!).

- **THE SHIT STORM SCHEDULE:** This is someone who has a schedule that's all over the place. You might need to do this schedule weekly to get your exercise in. Find 3 days where you can head out for a walk, head to the gym or go to a class that fits your schedule. Anything to get you moving and free your mind. I understand having a crazy schedule work wise can be nuts. But this should make it all that more important to make time for yourself to unwind. You might think it's more of a hassle to find time for yourself, but let me guarantee you one thing. You will appreciate it. Your body will appreciate it. Your work production will appreciate it. If you are a manager reading this, allow your staff to hit the gym at lunch. It actually improves work production and lowers the stress in the workplace. Go figure. #JustSaying

   - LITTLE MONSTERS: If you have kids and find it hard to workout, perhaps finding a gym that offers child care would be a good fit. If you can't find one, see if a family member or friend who supports your new fitness goals would be willing to watch your kids for an hour. You can also try getting fit at home with your kids! Find a DVD workout program that is realistic for you at this current time. Get your kids to take part or if they are too young, keep them by you with toys to keep them occupied. If they are old enough, get them to take part in some exercise! Why not start them young and get them in the habit? I know, some of you reading this are moms... Are probably yelling at this book saying, "But the kids keep me so busy I don't have the energy". OK, have you tried focusing on your nutrition and taking time FOR YOURSELF to be active or get out of the house? Remember, I don't mean only lifting weights. This could be you grabbing the bike and heading out for a half hour while someone watches the kids. Bringing the dogs for a walk. Free your brain!

– TRAVEL A LOT FOR WORK: Do your research on the hotel you are staying in and see if they have a gym. Get up 30 minutes before you usually would to get in quick workout before you start your day. Can be as simple as walking on the treadmill! Hate the treadmill? Maybe make it a point to get out and walk around to see the new city you are in. Worst case scenario, bring some gear with you when you travel. Best piece of equipment that will fit in your luggage, TRX. You can do loads of different exercises with this rig. No, I don't get royalties for mentioning TRX! It's good shit and I'm suggesting something that can help you! If you don't want to bring anything with you, do 30 push-ups, 30 squats, 30 lunges, 30 dips off a chair and :30 seconds of high knees. Carry on.

More and more of society operate what I call 'Desk Jockey' positions. This is where you sit in a desk all day. You are locked in for over 8 hours a day, staring at a screen with more than likely bad ergonomics and posture. You complain about lower back pain, headaches and low energy. Your boss won't give you your lunch break to workout. Lame. If you aren't able to escape your cubical to better your health, (which might I add helps with work production and better team moral...) you can do simple things to keep your body from locking up. Set a timer on your phone or email reminder to set every 30 minutes. When the timer goes off, get up and do 10 body weight squats. Next time the timer goes off, walk down the hallway. Goes off again, drop and do 10 push ups. All things that can be done while in your sandbox. Another suggestion if your supervisor allows it, sit on an exercise ball instead of a chair. This forces you to sit up properly and engage your core. An adjustable desk, go from seated to standing. If you have a really cool boss with a sweet budget, treadmill desk! Yep, walk and type at the same time.

It's important to find something you enjoy doing. When people feel forced into certain things, their chances of success fall because they lose interest. Maybe it's kickboxing, step class, floor hockey, soccer, whatever! Do something 3 days a week that gets you moving instead of sitting. Do something fun and keeps you interested.

GET SHIT DONE

My half sister Natasha. She couldn't be bothered with lifting weights. However, she LOVES Zumba! She does Zumba 3 days a week, loves it and goes every time. Not to mention she is a pretty good salsa dancer! I'm the other way around, I couldn't be bothered with Zumba, also doesn't help that I have 2 left feet (not really...I have a left foot and right foot...). She found her sweet spot, Zumba!

I have another client Reena who loves to come to the club to see me. No, not because I make her lift weights or because she clearly misses me (duh). She comes in for some one on one boxing. That's what keeps her motivated to come in. It's her sanity and escape. She feels excited to come in and energized when she leaves. Or at least that's what she tells me. (ha!) If I made the entire session weight lifting, she probably wouldn't be as excited. Just like cardio, don't ask Reena to walk on a treadmill. What gets her going? Walking the dogs!

I love pushing myself to lift weights or as I say... Pick shit up and put shit down. There is something invigorating about being able to lift heavy and push myself. Then there is Muay Thai. Nothing better than throwing around some heavy kicks, punches, sharp elbows and knees! Something about being mentally locked in and shut off from the world. There are no phones or televisions around to distract me. Let's face it, if there were distractions, I'd be getting knocked out weekly!

Different strokes for different folks! Find something active that works for you and keeps you coming back for more. If you're constantly dragging ass, maybe it's time to look into something new. The fitness industry is always growing and evolving, there is bound to be something out there you will want to try. I just drove by a strip mall by my house and noticed another 'fitness' business going up with a unique twist. I'm telling you, new places are popping up on the daily! Look around and try them out. You'd be surprised at what you might strike your fancy.

"SOMETIMES YOU JUST GOTTA GET SHIT DONE!"

– ASHLEY MATHIEU

CHAPTER 4:
THE HELP

If you read the last chapter and catch yourself thinking, "I want to go to the gym but I have no idea what I'm doing". That's OK! This chapter I will cover how to hire a trainer and what to look for. There are certain things you need to pay attention to in order to avoid red flags. Hiring a trainer isn't as easy as, "Oh you say you're certified, cool let's start tomorrow".

Being in the fitness industry for over 10 years as an athlete and fitness professional, I have come across a lot of shitty trainers. No, not solely based on skill. Some develop an ego that even a jackhammer can't break down. They think they are the best thing out there, everyone else is less than them and feel the need to puff their chest out. Then there are the people who take an online course and think they can train anyone and everyone with little to no experience in the gym. Don't get me wrong, you have to

GET SHIT DONE

start somewhere in any career, but thinking you are a super hero trainer straight out of the gate is a little much. Put your cape away, open a book, work with other trainers and develop a humble attitude. When I first started training people on my own, I was buried in books trying to learn. When I got my butt in a big box club, I asked a few trainers to shadow them to see their style and how maybe I could incorporate new things into my style of training. I would work out with different trainers and try new things. One of the biggest takeaways from doing this. Keeping an open mind. Never close yourself off. Accept criticism. Something I always teach my students.

FOR THE CONSUMER

If you are looking to hire help, these are some things I want you to do and things I want you to look for. Start by researching the market. Find out the rates. Ask how long the sessions are. What you get with those sessions. Payment plans and payment methods. The criteria of the trainer and establishment.

- If their method of payment is cash only, RUN. (Pay them and then they take off with your

money. Seen it one too many times) If you don't run, get a receipt and signature.
- If you are dealing with a private training studio, be prepared to pay a bit more as it's more of a private atmosphere. (Good for those not wanting distractions or are intimidated by gyms)
- Is the individual certified? Ask them from where and research it! Just because they say they are certified doesn't mean a whole lot. Is their certification recognized throughout the country, accepted by clubs looking to hire? (If their certification is from Joe Blows Online personal training, you might want to steer clear of that trainer. Just saying.)
- What's their background with physical fitness, life story and education? (Did they just jump into training because they couldn't find another job? You want a trainer who gives a shit, not one who's only doing it for a pay cheque)
- Are they planning on doing more upcoming training or courses? If so, which ones and why? (If they say they have learned everything there is to know about training. Red flag. Fitness industry is constantly growing and changing)
- Do they have YOUR interest at heart? (Are they just telling you what THEY want to do? Ignoring what your goals are? Red flag)

- Are they able to give you a picture of what you can expect from them program wise? (If the trainer can't give you an example of a simple periodization plan, walk away. They should be able to talk to you about a plan of action and possible changes down the road)
- Are they charging you for a consult? (If the trainer is charging you to meet you, think about it. They are charging you, the potential client, who could possibly spend a few hundred or few thousand dollars on them. Move on)
- Check the fine print on contracts. ALWAYS. (Don't get screwed)

When you sit down with a fitness professional, I want you to treat it like a job interview. Don't go into a club and hire anyone because they have a picture on the wall with a quick bio. I want you to blast them with questions and voice any concerns you have. When you go buy a car, do you not ask questions about the warranty, how things work and what ifs? When you are hiring an employee, do you not ask them questions to make sure you are bringing on a qualified individual to get the job done? Hiring a trainer is no different. Furthermore, if the trainer can't answer something, don't hold that against them. Not everyone knows the answer to everything. What you want to hear is, "I am not sure, but I will look into it and get back to you". That is what you want to hear. A trainer who isn't afraid to ask for help or a second opinion. Your body and your money is on the line. Interview them. I use to ask potential clients to go interview other trainers. Not because I was cocky. I did that because they would be unsure and instead of pressuring them to buy, I would tell them to compare what I have to offer versus others. That worked out well for me. Why? Because I was honest.

TO THE TRAINER

If you are a trainer reading this book, I hope the majority of you who are in the fitness industry are truly in it for the right reasons. I get a natural high from seeing clients progress and hit their goals. I hope you do too. Nothing more motivating than to see your client finish a chemo treatment and still show up to train. The client who is going through personal issues, shows up and you become the reason for the smile when they leave. The excitement after you see your client bend down and tie their shoe while standing for the first time in 5 years because they lost weight. The pumped up F**K YEAH moment that happens when your client smashes out chin ups for the first time. The high fives that get thrown around after your client tells you they need new pants because their current ones are falling off when walking down the street! Better yet, when your friends ask if you shit yourself your pants are so saggy!

Let's face it, when putting the mindset forward to becoming a trainer, you're not doing it for the money. If you are new and think you are going to make a six figure salary in the first year, good luck with that. I'm not trying to be a dick, I am being realistic. We do this job because we give a shit. We care about the clients. We care about health and we want to help. Case and point.

IF YOU ARE A TRAINER WITH THE FOLLOWING MINDSET:

- Doing it for dating purposes
- For a pay cheque
- Because you like to stare at yourself in the mirror
- This is a last resort before you go homeless
- Doesn't give a shit

You should probably look for a new career or change your mind set. You are ruining what it means to be a fitness professional and giving the rest of us a bad look.

SOME TIPS TO MY FITNESS PROFESSIONALS OUT THERE:

- Keep learning
- Stay interested
- Network with other health and fitness professionals
- Keep an open mind
- Never have an ego
- Have fun, laugh, be the reason your client had an awesome day
- Give. A. Shit.

I SAW A SHINY OBJECT...

There are a lot of really good people out there in the fitness industry who truly want to help. Like any industry, there are people who you may want to throat punch. Happens everywhere. You want to feel comfortable with the person, trust them and most importantly, not want to throat punch them! Interview a few trainers and see who you mesh with. At

GET SHIT DONE

the end of the day, it's your body you are trusting to them and your finances being put out. Be smart. Don't be in a rush. If you set out to find a trainer and don't feel a connection with anyone that you have met, keep searching.

"A PERSON WHO NEVER MADE A MISTAKE NEVER TRIED ANYTHING NEW"

– ALBERT EINSTEIN

CHAPTER 5:
FUELING YOUR BODY FOR SUCCESS

One of the largest parts of living a healthy lifestyle is being able to have a balanced diet. I don't even like using the word diet because it's been given such a negative tone thanks to media. Don't be freaked out when I use the word 'diet'.

What everyone needs to understand is that the food we put in our mouths is what fuels our bodies. If you are someone who eats a tonne of sweets, chances are your insulin levels are spiking which makes you hungry faster, more often, more tired and not to mention gain weight. Then there are the opposite people who simply don't eat because they think if they don't eat they will lose weight. Well, sorry to break the news to you... NOT eating will only stress your body out, leading it to either eat away at itself or store the food your slamming back. Then you run into metabolism, thyroid, adrenal and a bunch of other health issues.

Since I deal with everyone on an individual basis, I am not going to attach a 'meal plan' for everyone. Remember, we are not all the same. What I do for someone may not work for the next. However, what I can do is help YOU understand more about food!

- 1 gram of protein = 4 calories
- 1 gram of carbohydrates = 4 calories
- 1 gram of fat = 9 calories

TIP: On training days have meals with carbs before you work out and after. Non training days, only have carbs for breakfast. Rest of the meals have fats (10g – 14g) for your energy source.

When you are shopping for groceries, try and stick to whole foods. Foods that are fresh, not in can or come pre made. Make sure to wash your veggies and fruits before you eat them. Get all the grime off them! Just because the apples look shiny and yummy in the store, doesn't mean they are clean. How many times do you touch an apple to see if it's bruised and put it back? Get it?

GET $HIT DONE

While going the whole foods route, you are avoiding the chemical shit storm. Boxed, canned and bagged foods more often than not contain a lot of preservatives, chemicals and dyes. Not to mention genetically modified ingredients.

It's important to understand that yes, your grocery bill might be more expensive going the whole foods route. Eating healthy can get pricier than eating junk. Shop around, check flyers and make wise decisions. Another thing you can do is look at your useless spending habits. Are you buying tea and coffee every morning? Are you eating out for breakfast, lunch and dinner during the week instead of meal prepping? Are you a smoker spending a couple hundred dollars a month on smokes?

EXAMPLES OF WHOLE FOODS:

- Fruits
- Vegetables
- Proteins
- Nuts, seeds
- Healthy fats (no, margarine is not a healthy fat!)

Whole foods are pretty much anything that grows from the earth or runs around! Whole foods do not consist of pre made frozen dinners, chips, cookies or soft drinks! Cleaner you eat, the cleaner your body will run and the better mindset you will be in. Your body works in a continuous circle. Body, Mind, Soul. If you have a gas powered car, are you going to put diesel in it? No, because the car won't run properly and will break down. Just like your body does when you feed it shit. Remember that being healthy is not about what you look like on the outside, but your mind and soul. Everything works together.

Nutrition Facts
Valeur nutritive
Per 1 Cup (250mL) / pour 1 tasse (250 mL)

Amount Teneur	% Daily Value % valeur quotidienne
Calories / Calories 80	
Fat/Lipides 0 g	0 %
Saturated / saturés 0 g	0 %
+ Trans / trans 0 g	
Cholesterol / Cholestérol 0 mg	0 %
Sodium / Sodium 10 mg	0 %
Potassium / Potassium 250 mg	7 %
Carbohydrates /Glucides 19 g	6 %
Fibre / Fibres less than 1g	3 %
Sugars / Sucres 16 g	
Protein / Protéines less than 1g	
Vitamin A/ Vitamine A	0 %
Vitamin C / Vitamine C	100 %
Calcium / Calcium	0 %
Iron / Fer	2 %

When looking at putting together your daily meals, pay attention to the food labels. Not just how many calories are in the item but also for the small print everyone decides not to read. The ingredients. Once you read the ingredient label on many processed food boxes, you will be amazed at the amount of chemicals and junk. Thus, hopefully steering you away from buying it! Start reading all your labels! #SorryNotSorry for when you start getting grossed out!

You want to pay attention to the serving size, fats, sodium, carbohydrates, sugars and protein. You want know that you are getting your proper 'macros' in every meal. Macros are your proteins, fats and carbohydrates. If you don't pay attention, you could either be putting yourself in a deficit or over eating. It's important to understand if your body is getting enough fuel.

FUN FACT: YOUR STOMACH IS THE SIZE OF YOUR FIST. STOP SHOVING DOWN MASSIVE PLATES OF FOOD!

Some basic tips:

- Fats: Stick to under 12g per meal
- Sodium: Daily intake should not be more than 1500mg
- Carbohydrates: Try to stay under 40g per meal
- Protein: Try staying around 30-40g per meal

- **SODA DRINKERS:** Try and knock off the soda. Just because you drink 'diet' soda, doesn't make it any better. Diet soda is what I call cancer in a can. Filled with chemicals. Why are you putting chemicals in your body? If you are someone who drinks pop on a regular basis, try taking down your intake bit by bit instead of going cold turkey. You will go through withdrawals if you go cold turkey. Example, you drink about 8 sodas a week. You find you drink them mostly at work. Great, your new goal is to eliminate the soda at home. At home stick with water, lemon water, green tea, natural stuff! If you slowly eliminate it, this may make it easier. If you try cold turkey, your rate of going back to it is a lot higher! Remember this word... BALANCE! But hey, if you are the type of person that can handle the extreme change, do it!

- **SWEET TOOTH:** If you always have dessert after every dinner, try doing it every second day. Take a step away for a bit to let the craving where off. Many times it's a mental game because of a habit you have set over time. Your brain knows the pattern and sets itself to understanding when it's getting a treat.

What I do for my sweet tooth. I take half a cup of plain Greek yogurt with some chocolate natural whey protein. Mix that up and enjoy! It's not exactly cheese cake, but it satisfies me! Sometimes I will sip on some tea, have a coffee or chew on some gum. For those with a bigger craving, look into journaling your thoughts into a book. Write down what you are craving, why you are craving it, how you will feel when you are eating it, how you will feel right after you eat it and how you will feel 1 hour after that!

- CARBOHYDRATES: Carbs are not a BAD thing. You need carbs for performance both in sport and brain function! However, over consuming them while doing NOTHING to burn them off isn't a good idea. If you're eating 200g of carbs in a day, you better damn well be getting a good workout in! Chances are you probably eat a good chunk of fat and sugars as well. One easy way to help with weight loss is eat your starches before 2pm. The rest of the day consume veggies, protein and a bit of healthy fats. Measure how many carbs you are eating, again using the nutrition labels. If it's rice, use a measuring cup. If it's bread or a wrap, start understanding how many carbs are in a slice so you can make better decisions when on the road. If you know by 2pm you have consumed 100g of carbs, you should probably lay off the rest of the day and stick to proteins, fats and greens. Even more so if you are not active.

- PROTEIN: Protein won't make you look like a man (if you are a female reader) or make you fat. Protein helps repair and build muscle, but also important for your tendons, cartilage, bones and blood. If you are working out, you need to consume protein! I don't care if you get it via a vegan diet or eat every animal on the planet, just get it in you! If you're not eating it, don't complain about not getting rid of flabby arms, being tired, sore and your strength not improving. Some people will ask, "How much should I have in a day?". Well to answer that, everyone is different! There are many philosophies out there discussing how much someone should consume. Honestly, find your sweet spot with how your body breaks it down.

Let's do an example and some math! Are you doing it for weight loss or putting on size? You can tinker around with it. Start with taking .75 X (your weight). Example, I will do .75 X 155lbs = 116.25g of protein per day. If I eat 4 meals a day, that means each meal should have 29g of protein in them. You could do more, like .85 or 1.0 per point of body weight. Again, do with what your body is happy with. If you find going 1g X 1lbs is making you bloated or tired, then maybe hack it down to .85g x 1lbs. For me personally, if I have a meal with too much protein, I will be bloated, tired and feel heavy. Red meat also destroys me.

GET $HIT DONE

- **FATS:** Stop being afraid of the word FAT! Fats don't make you FAT! They are essential for the body, hormone production, transportation of vitamins throughout the body, healthier skin and key for sport performance. You need good fat to get rid of bad fat! Drives me nuts when I hear people tell me they aren't eating fat because they are trying to lose weight. Mind. Blown. Obviously if you are eating deep fried food all day, that's bad fat and you will gain weight! Not rocket science. So don't take this part of the book and say you could eat a large amount of deep fried chicken wings! That's BAD FAT! When consuming fats, make sure they are healthy fats and in moderation. Some good examples of fats are nuts, coconut oil, olive oil, nut butters, grass fed butter, avocados etc... Fats are high in caloric value, so check the nutrition label before you tell me you just ate an entire bag of almonds from Costco!

- **FRUITS:** Way too many people are afraid of fruit because they contain sugar. Yes, fruits do have sugar. Some are higher in the glycemic index than others. So in other terms, some fruits contain more sugar than others and some can spike your insulin faster than others. YOU need to educate yourself on the glycemic index. Why? Do you have a family members with diabetes? Insulin issues? Have you been told to watch your sugar intake? This is why you need to pay attention. You need to understand which fruits to avoid so you don't piss off your body and make it spike, crash and go in a vicious cycle.

EXAMPLE OF FRUITS THAT ARE LOWER IN THE GLYCEMIC INDEX ARE:

- Blueberries
- Raspberries
- Blackberries
- Apples
- Kiwi

EXAMPLES OF FRUITS THAT ARE HIGHER IN THE GLYCEMIC INDEX. YOU MAY WANT TO AVOID FRUITS LIKE THESE IF YOU HAVE ISSUES WITH SUGAR:

- Canned fruits with syrup
- Pineapple
- Watermelon
- Raisins
- Cantaloupe

GET SHIT DONE

RANDOM POINT: TRY PUTTING CINNAMON ON YOUR FRUIT, HELPS WITH INSULIN SENSITIVITY!

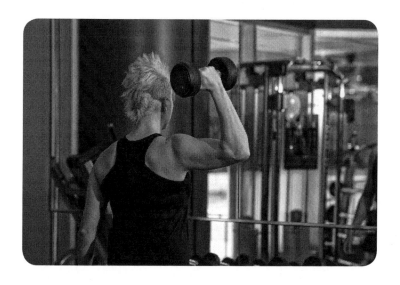

Lastly, don't stress out about food. If you are making good food choices and not over eating, you are already on the right path. This is a starting point. If you don't read things (food labels) and stop paying attention, that's when the unwanted weight gain creeps in and health issues pop up. Start off slow, get the body used to the changes to avoid cravings and freak outs! It's important to remember the word 'balance' and understand it's OK to have a cookie or go out for lunch with friends. It's all about moderation and making smart decisions. Don't limit yourself and eliminate everything from your diet. Telling yourself you CAN'T have something will only end up making you crave it. So if you have done well for 3 days and one day you see a cookie you want, eat it! Yep, I just said eat the cookie! If you are someone that does 'cheat days', make sure you alternate the day so your body doesn't get use to having something deep fried on Saturday at 5pm! Your body is smarter than you think so you should probably confuse it!

"HAVE A HEALTHY BALANCE IN LIFE AND YOU WILL BE HAPPIER THAN BEING 100% ANAL ABOUT EVERYTHING!"

– ASHLEY MATHIEU

CHAPTER 6:
SUPPLEMENTS – DO YOU NEED THEM?

When starting with a client I always get them to answer a lengthy questionnaire. One of the questions asks if they take any supplements. If I see a list of supplements on the sheet written down, I am going to ask why. Many people over supplement themselves and end up wasting a lot of money.

DID YOU KNOW?

- Vitamins A,D,E,K are fat soluble vitamins. Taking too much can lead to negative side effects.
- All others are water soluble, what your body doesn't absorb is secreted through urine.

GET $HIT DONE

- Consult your doctor, Naturopath or Holistic Practitioner prior to consuming supplements.
- Are you taking medications? Consult with a doctor before ingesting other supplements as they could have a negative reaction.

Don't be freaked out about supplements. Supplements are here for a reason, but be smart about how and WHY you are taking them. Let me break it down in the simplest form I can think of, straight out of my blog.

LET'S START OUT WITH THOSE WHO ARE FRESH OFF THE COUCH:

First thing you need to work on or build into your lifestyle is NUTRITION! You need to make sure you are eating enough to power your body throughout your regular workday and fitness program. If you aren't eating enough, you will get tired, your body will start eating itself and you will be one angry S.O.B! Start with cleaning up your diet and taking on a REALISTIC (there it is...) training program. Do that for the first month or two and see how your body is reacting. If your body hates you, please keep reading for more advice...

ASHLEY MATHIEU

SOMEONE WHO IS HITTING THE GYM FOR LIFESTYLE AND HAS BEEN FOR A WHILE:

This is the crowd where I get tonnes of questions from. "Should I be taking supplements to get better results"? Some of the supplements they are talking about are BCAA's, Pre-Workouts, multi vitamin packs, caffeine pills, fat loss pills, protein powders etc...

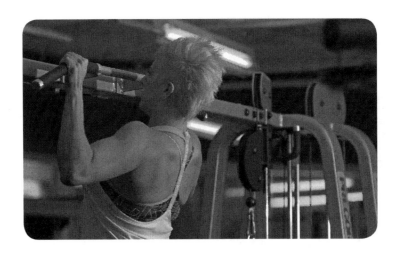

I would be looking at nutrition and progressive overload... Are you eating properly for your goals, lifestyle and training? Are you changing up your workout routines enough to appropriately avoid the plateau and bring your body to a new level? More often than not, nutrition and programming are usually the issue as to why the results have stopped. It's not that you need to buy hundreds of dollars of supplements, it's that you need to sit down with someone who's a professional to pick you apart. Doing this, they can give you more accurate pointers and give you better natural results.

ATHLETE OR SERIOUS GYM GO-ERRRRR!

Here is where things can get a bit more involved and also a lot stickier. From a personal stand point, I try and get all my fuel from food. I'll drink BCAA's during my workout very rarely, if ever, unless I am taking part in a rigorous training program. Some people need that added 'umph' and require taking in certain supplements. In most cases, high level athletes are unable to get everything in via food, so they need that added edge with supplements. They can assist with keeping your body fueled longer, help with recovery, muscle growth, endurance etc... Athletes are exhausting their bodies, thus needing some added support for themselves (ATP)... For an average Joe working out, no, supplements aren't needed unless medically specified!

Lastly, please don't fall into the trap of buying a bunch of powders and supplements from a friend who decided to start selling some product for extra money on the side, who themselves know nothing about nutrition and aren't a fitness professional. Just saying. I understand people want to make more money, but buying products from someone who isn't educated and repeating what someone else told them isn't the smartest thing to do. Be smart about where you get your products from. I get my supplements straight from my Naturopath or from a natural food store that carries high end products. I spend the time researching that I am taking and if I can't find the answers, I ask someone.

Majority of people are deficient in something. But again, before you go popping pills, go to your doctor to see what your body needs. Better safe than sorry.

"SLOW YOUR THOUGHTS DOWN AND GET OUT OF YOUR HEAD. ELIMINATE THE SELF DESTRUCTIVE MIND AND STEP FORWARD INTO CLARITY."

– ASHLEY MATHIEU

CHAPTER 7:
STRETCH YOURSELF

Everyone needs to stretch. Simple. Whether you are on your feet all day or sit in a desk. Stretching improves your mobility, your range of motion, posture, injury prevention and helps aid in stress management. It's not rocket science that doing nothing will make you stiff and give you unwanted aches. Not stretching = you stiff. Not stretching can be one of the leading factors in you hitting a plateau with weight training. I'm not saying you need to start yoga! But yes, Yoga will defiantly help! If you can't get to a class for whatever reason, there are plenty of television stations and online websites where you can find free yoga to do from home. Or better yet, sit on the floor while you watch the news and STRETCH!

There are a few forms of stretching and mobility exercises:

- *Static Stretching:* These are stretches that you hold in place. These stretches are better off done after a workout or done while watching TV!
- *Dynamic Stretching:* Movement based stretching. Example of this would be doing circles with your arms, swinging your leg left to right, rotating your trunk, high knees etc... This will raise the heart rate, get your circulation going, allow the synovial fluid to release and your muscles to get ready for activity. This is done before you workout and also during if you need.
- *Foam Rolling:* Yes, that lovely tube you roll on, its good shit! This tube you see people awkwardly rolling on helps with myofascial release. Grinding out those stubborn knots in the muscle. Not only is it like giving yourself a deep tissue massage, it helps with circulation, range of motion and recovery. This can be done before, during and after physical activity.

Stretching should not only be done around exercise, but also in the morning before you start your day, at work or at night when watching TV (notice how this is the second time I am telling you to do it in front of the TV). It doesn't take much time to stretch, again it's making the time. Stretching is a good stress reliever, which is why I mentioned yoga. Being able to disconnect from the world and really unwind is important. Today's society is wired to electronics and overly stressed out.

Not going to lie. I use to HATE stretching! I found it boring and a waste of time. It wasn't until shit started hitting the fan in life that I actually appreciated shutting my brain off. I thank Todd for that one. I saw him doing crazy head stands, covered in tattoos and lifting heavy shit. He would always ask me when I was going to do one of his classes. My classic answer was always telling him I'd go sometime soon. Lies. Straight up lies! But, I knew I had to do one of his classes, mainly so he would stop asking. One day I stepping into one of his hot yoga classes. He is the reason I developed my respect for yoga. I still don't understand how he can stand on one leg and do some pretzel shit and not fall over... Insane. You win Todd... You win! Respect.

Back to why I like yoga... It taught me how awesome it is to disconnect, quiet my mind and centre myself. There is something very spiritual about yoga and being able to connect with yourself. If you've never done yoga, you probably have no idea what I'm talking about. Go, you will see what I mean.

GET $HIT DONE

Then there are the obvious points, like better sport performance, flexibility and strength gains. So get out there, find a yoga joint and try a class! You won't regret it.

SIDE BAR: TAKE AN HOUR A DAY AND GET OFF THE INTERNET, OFF THE PHONE AND AWAY FROM THE TV. YOUR BODY AND BRAIN WILL THANK YOU.

"BE WHO YOU ARE AND NOT WHAT
PEOPLE WANT YOU TO BE…"

– ASHLEY MATHIEU

CHAPTER 8:
AVOID THE MEDIA & HYPE

N ow here is a chapter where I am going to be very straight forward. Shocking, I know! How can I possibly be any more straight forward than I have already been?

Point blank, the media is the best at creating a shit storm when it comes to promoting weight loss products. They are very good at putting together engaging commercials, sweet looking ads in the magazines you stare at while you wait to check out of the grocery store and badass billboards along the highway. I might get some flak for this chapter, but hey... I am speaking the truth.

One of the scariest things I saw when traveling through Los Angeles, CA was seeing all the billboards for a certain type of 'weight loss' surgery. I couldn't believe how many signs I saw along the highway, it was insane! I understand the obesity rate in the US is high, but... What. The. Eff. People who are not educated about exercise and nutrition probably read those signs as a relief and life saver. Yes, some people need more extreme measures than just what they are eating and how they exercise. Putting it out to the masses like it's a flu shot... Not right. Actually makes me pretty upset and frustrated to see this is how society has decided to treat obesity. End rant.

Tea. Skinny Tea. Diet Tea. Buying a special tea that claims you will lose weight. Awesome! Of course you are going to lose some weight. You want to know why!? Because you are going to shit yourself, THAT'S WHY! Do you know how many people ask me about these teas? "Drink this tea in the morning and have this one before bed"... Yeah, so you can shit your pants off while at work or as soon as you wake up (hopefully you make it to the bathroom!) in the morning. No filter. Honestly people... Tea?

If you are looking at cleansing your system, eat whole foods. Avoid eating junk and processed crap. On another note, if you're backed up, sure... Drink the tea! Just make sure to map out the nearest bathroom. If you already have a sensitive system, you should probably avoid the tea all together. Don't forget to bring another pair of pants to work. In all seriousness, if you really want to try a colon cleanse and all that nasty jazz, try getting a colonic. I have had a few friends who have done it. They liked it and actually learned a lot from it. Have I done one? Nope. Haven't 'manned up' yet. Lastly, if you have digestive issues, go see your doctor.

Weight loss pills. Another topic clients enjoy asking me about. Listen people, weight loss doesn't happen overnight. It takes time, effort and balance. Taking a pill in hopes you will lose the weight fast while still eating junk won't work. Taking over the counter thermogenics might be more harmful to your body than you think. There may be things inside the pills your body doesn't agree with. This can lead to headaches, low energy, stomach issues, rashes, respiratory issues and so on. Don't get me wrong, there are some natural thermogenics out there that can help aid in weight loss with a healthy diet, but consult with your doctor or holistic practitioner before you start popping pills. Or better yet, research what you are about to put in your body.

If you read something about a, "NEW revolutionary weight loss product" please run, flip the page or change the channel. Unfortunately we have celebrities blasting out promotions for stuff like this. Stop buying into the hype. You are wasting your money. Here's an idea, next time you want to buy some gimmick product, send me the money instead to puregritfitness@gmail.com. I'll do something awesome with it. Promise. But seriously, stop thinking, "OK this product looks way more legit than the last one"... Because it's NOT! Same shit, different day. I don't care what famous doctor on television says it works. I don't care what magazine says it's the new best thing. Trust your gut when you think something is too good to be true. If it looks like shit, smells like shit, it's probably shit.

Like I've spoken about already, find your balance with food and activity. That is the best form of medical insurance! Food is your fuel, food is your weight loss pill, food is what gets you from point A to point B and what keeps you burning!

"WHY SETTLE FOR BEING LESS THAN YOU ARE
WHEN YOU CAN BE ALL KINDS OF AWESOME"

– ASHLEY MATHIEU

CHAPTER 9:
I'LL SHUT UP NOW

So by now you have read all the chapters or at least I hope you did. You have either come to the conclusion that living a happy and healthy lifestyle isn't that hard or that you have some serious decisions to make. It doesn't need to be done overnight so don't stress over it. You don't need to give up everything you thought you did, just make adjustments. I hope you have realized by now that the key to a happy and healthy lifestyle is BALANCE! If you are completely new to this whole health thing, that's OK! Think of this read as your first step. If you are someone that tried to get on the health wagon but fell off, hopefully this information has given you some insight to help you jump back on and kick some ass! If you are someone that needs to change direction career wise or life wise, take it one step at a time.

One thing I always recommend to clients is to create a journal. Log what you are eating so you can keep yourself accountable, keep track of your exercise to see your progression and write down your mood. The times you feel down, feel like binging on food or when you don't have someone to talk to, write it down! If you find yourself binging in these situations, get your journal out and write down stuff down. Don't read it... Just write and a week later read it! You may find a common trend and find your triggers. Other reason is, your mind might be so clouded that if you read it right away, you still won't understand. Give it time and revisit it later.

Leading a healthy lifestyle is always work! There is an overload of information everyday on what is healthy and what is no longer healthy... Don't get caught up in the hype. Keep the balance and simplicity of health in line and you will be just fine! Again, when you think something is too good to be true, it more than likely probably is!

In terms of those of you who may be considering changing your career, be smart. Make sure you map everything out right before you take the leap. I'm a pretty bad example of that, I just jumped and put myself into a corner. Only way out of a corner is…. well straight ahead! My plan wasn't concrete, I made a split second decision to leave because I was about to go postal (figure of speech). Lucky for me it's turned out very well. But if I could suggest anything to any of you who are contemplating leaving, think it through. If you can take a year no pay from your job, with it guaranteed when you come back, do it. This way if your plans fall through, you have your old job still kicking. If you don't have that option, make the necessary steps to make your jump worth it. Never take your foot off the gas. Never let hurdles stop you. Never keep your mind in the box, start thinking outside the box. Never ever put limitations on yourself.

Live life. Be healthy. Be happy. Smile. Help others. Thank you and hope you will join the journey of awesome! Now go on… Get Started… And…
GET. SHIT. DONE

ACKNOWLEDGEMENTS

Alright, time to thank some people in my life who have helped me get to where I am today. Of course I have to start off with my parents. Let's face it, if it wasn't for Maria and Gordon, I wouldn't be here! Thank you for always putting up with my shit and supporting me during my most random and insane moments in life. I know I am not the most straight edged kid, nor do I ever want to be. Thank you for letting me be me. Also to my family members who have learned to adapt to my madness.

To my brother in law Ender Atay. Thanks for snapping sweet photos of my ever so delicate face for this book.

To my closest friends who have stuck by me since my teen years, thank you Mathew Mcrae, Erik Turcot and Tanya Dunn for always being there and supporting me through everything I've gone through. Having friends who you can count on can be tough.

The kind that knows when something is up, picks up the phone after months of not communicating and checks in. The kind of buddies who you can count on to shoot the shit and set you straight when you need it. Thanks stooges!

To my coaches Alain Sylvestre, Michael Fisher, Sacha Hijazi, Alain Moussi and Stephan Roy for testing me, pushing me and having a place to go to relieve some unwanted stress on the mats and in the ring. I truly know that martial arts is what helped me get through many of my obstacles in life.

Every single one of my clients. You guys inspire me every day. Whether you were coming to see me for weight loss, stress, performance or post medical ... You have all played a very active role in what I do today and continue to do tomorrow. Thank you for being awesome. Thank you for putting your trust in me and not throat punching me.

Mike Robinson. The man of steel. Thank you for not only supporting me the last few years, but also taking me under your wing sort to speak. For believing in me and being a part of my rollercoaster ride. For taking risks with a woman at the time you didn't completely know. For giving me tough love, listening to me, respecting me, taking a risk and always being there to give sounds advice when I need it. Honestly, thank you. No, this doesn't mean you get a hug. We are still rubbing elbows.

I must thank wordpress.com . If it wasn't for wordpress, I wouldn't have been able to reach thousands of people with my random blogs! Thanks wordpress for hosting my blog and allowing a shit like me to express myself!

MY EAST COAST CREW! Can't forget you guys! Let's be real here, I met most, if not all of you loaded in a pub. Best ever! Christina Weagle and Shawna Theriault. 10 years later, here we are! Thanks for supporting me from a far, letting me take part in your lives on a personal stand point and always being real. Nova Scotia, you are like my second home.

Anytime Fitness for allowing me into the brand! Thank you for letting me be a part of the purple tribe and being super cool! Best franchise of life. For real. Chuck Runyon, your hair is pretty epic. Coming from me, that's a big deal (ha). To the crew at corporate for being a bunch of awesome. Yep, just a bunch of awesome.

To anyone who commented, 'liked' or 'hearted' anything on my Instagram, Twitter, Snapchat, Youtube, Periscope and any other social media I have out there. Thanks. You're good shit.

Francis, Bill, Jeff and Jimmy. Thanks for the fun times and trusting me to be your co-pilot. Martin, thanks for giving me the go ahead to travel all over and do crazy stuff. Paulina, thanks for not hitting me with the taser and giving me the 'ride for 5'. Sly, for being my workplace father figure and being there to shoot the breeze. Not to mention take me under your wing and teach me a thing or two :)

To all my club members. Thanks for joining. Thanks for working out. Thanks for not trashing my gym. Thanks for bringing in all your baked goods you can't eat.

Lastly, to every single one of you who has been following me on my journey. Words cannot express how much of an awesome feeling it is to have people from all over the world supporting you. Your support keeps me fueled to keep learning, keep inspiring and motivating people every single day. If it wasn't for every single one of you, I wouldn't have been inspired to write this book. Thank you. All of you. Seriously.

Oh. Thanks for reading.

ASHLEY'S PICKS

Here are some supplements and reading material I love! Clean and good quality stuff.

SUPPLEMENTS:

www.aor.ca
I use their vitamin B complex, Adrenal supplement, vitamin C and glutamine powder.

www.restorativeformulations.com
Adaptogen (for adrenal support)
and Adrenal PX Balance

www.kyolic.com
Immune shield

ASHLEY MATHIEU

SPORT SUPPLEMENTS:

www.hardmagnum.com
Love their chocolate whey isolate!

www.optimumnutrition.com
Mocha Cappuccino Protein Energy powder

www.beyondyourself.ca
BCAA powder

READING MATERIAL:

www.mobilitywod.com
Dr. Kelly Starrett is the shit! Get his book 'Becoming A Supple Leopard'

www.cleaneatingmag.com
Awesome site for meal ideas.

www.thugkitchen.com
Hilarious and amazing cook book!

GET SHIT DONE

WORKOUT EQUIPMENT MUST HAVE'S:

www.yogatuneup.com
Therapy balls and DVD for mobility work.

www.trxtraining.com
Training system you can travel with.

www.thestick.com
More mobility gear to keep you from being stiff!

Your Journal

YOUR GOALS

Date: _____

Goal: _____

Why: _____

Date to be completed: _____

Did you complete it? Yes or No?
Explain how this Yes or No feels:

_____

_____

_____

_____

_____

_____

Date: _____

Goal: _____

Why: _____

Date to be completed: _____

Did you complete it? Yes or No?
Explain how this Yes or No feels:

_____

_____

_____

_____

_____

_____

_____

Date: _____

Goal: _____

Why: _____

Date to be completed: _____

Did you complete it? Yes or No?
Explain how this Yes or No feels:

_____

_____

_____

_____

_____

_____

_____

Date: _____

Goal: _____

Why: _____

Date to be completed: _____

Did you complete it? Yes or No?
Explain how this Yes or No feels:

_____

_____

_____

_____

_____

_____

_____

Date: _____

Goal: _____

Why: _____

Date to be completed: _____

Did you complete it? Yes or No?
Explain how this Yes or No feels:

_____

_____

_____

_____

_____

_____

Date: _____

Goal: _____

Why: _____

Date to be completed: _____

Did you complete it? Yes or No?
Explain how this Yes or No feels:

_____

_____

_____

_____

_____

_____

_____

Date: _____

Goal: _____

Why: _____

Date to be completed: _____

Did you complete it? Yes or No?
Explain how this Yes or No feels:

_____

_____

_____

_____

_____

_____

_____

Date: _____

Goal: _____

Why: _____

Date to be completed: _____

Did you complete it? Yes or No?
Explain how this Yes or No feels:

_____

_____

_____

_____

_____

_____

_____

Date: _____

Goal: _____

Why: _____

Date to be completed: _____

Did you complete it? Yes or No?
Explain how this Yes or No feels:

_____

_____

_____

_____

_____

_____

_____

Date: _____

Goal: _____

Why: _____

Date to be completed: _____

Did you complete it? Yes or No?
Explain how this Yes or No feels:

_____

_____

_____

_____

_____

_____

_____

Date: _____

Goal: _____

Why: _____

Date to be completed: _____

Did you complete it? Yes or No?
Explain how this Yes or No feels:

_____

_____

_____

_____

_____

_____

_____

Made in the USA
Columbia, SC
05 November 2017